I0440415

# Fun Ways To Do Pushups in One Minute (For Dummies)

(And yes for everyone else too !)

You will start off as a Novice and come out to be an expert.

by-

## ASHUTOSH TIWARI

Copyright © 2015 ASHUTOSH TIWARI

All rights reserved.

ISBN:1508933251
ISBN-13:9781508933250

# DEDICATION

Foremost this book is being dedicated to all those people(dummies) out there who say they do not have time to exercise. This book is been written keeping in mind that the readers are totally dummies and who just give excuses for not being able to exercise. This book dedicates to all those lazy people who want to have some sort of exercise but could not manage time in their daily routine. It guides them having some easy, funny and not so much time consuming ways to do pushups so that they no more could be able to complain about the time.

Just mind to give yourself 1 minute and you can call your workout to be 1 minute workout. Is not that cool? Yes, surely it is.

So all the lazy folks out there ! Come and lets have some fun ways to do pushups while reading this book.


Disclaimer :- This book is seriously for those who do not have time in their daily routine.

# CONTENTS

# DEDICATION

Foremost this book is being dedicated to all those people(dummies) out there who say they do not have time to exercise. This book is been written keeping in mind that the readers are totally dummies and who just give excuses for not being able to exercise. This book dedicates to all those lazy people who want to have some sort of exercise but could not manage time in their daily routine. It guides them having some easy, funny and not so much time consuming ways to do pushups so that they no more could be able to complain about the time.

Just mind to give yourself 1 minute and you can call your workout to be 1 minute workout. Is not that cool? Yes, surely it is.

So all the lazy folks out there ! Come and lets have some fun ways to do pushups while reading this book.

Disclaimer :- This book is seriously for those who do not have time in their daily routine.

# CONTENTS

# ACKNOWLEDGMENTS

In this section I want to acknowledge all those folks(including you) who have given this book their precious time of their so called busy schedule.

Last but not the least, I would like to thank myself because once in a while was also like you giving excuses in doing exercise. So, all the dummies out there lets have an awesome time( only you and me) in doing some of the most interesting ways to do pushups.

# PREFACE

I was just sitting on my desk, which is when I thought to why not share my experiences on pushups with you. I too had a same mentality that I do get time for exercise. It was just a pretty lame excuse.

This book is been written to just to start yourself to do exercise. I mean it, this will help. On the other hand, it will keep you fit. It talks all about pushups. This book is just been written to ensure oneself that, the next time I will not give excuses for not exercising.

I have been doing pushups while I was in 10th grade. So, it's not a big deal. Just give yourself one minute.

# FOREWORD

This book is all about pushups that is how to find some time from your busy schedule for exercising. It tells you why do we need to do pushups. This book is seriously for those who just complain that they do not have time from their routine and want to exercise.

After reading this book, you will think that how stupid I was that I used to complain of not finding just 1 minute of mine to give to exercising. This book lays emphasis upon the variety of pushups one can do. Pushups are just a great deed for your body. After 2-3 week you will be able to draw changes from your body. It will help you to keep you in shape by just giving 1 minute from 24 hours. Isn't that interesting? Yes it is !

This book is full of fun ways to do pushups with me and just trust me it is not that tough. After finishing this book you can become a self made expert on pushups. Teach your friends and colleagues what pushups can do to your body in just one minute.

Fun Ways To Do Pushups

# 1. LETS BEGIN(DAY 1)

I would not start the usual way of saying that you have to wake up early, or you have to cut down on media. Feel free to do anything you want. It's just that one has to have a balance among all the things. Please feel free to carry on with your daily routine. For all the readers(including you) those have not tried yet and those who have tried, it is all normal for you to follow.

Let's start with the basic. Since this is your first day, give a deep breath and just have in mind that I am going to start exercising. Really, it's not that tough. You just have to keep in mind that I will and I have to.

Just give yourself 1 minute. It could be just before taking a shower or till your bathing water gets warm. Or simply if you are waiting for your food to get cooked in a microwave, instead of just standing ideal and watching the timer, just do some exercise which will benefit you and you only. Stand against a wall with both your hands shoulder length apart touching the wall while keeping your body straight touching the ground. Make an inclined position. Lower your body half way down and then move backwards keeping your body straight.

Do this 5 times. Now you can carry on with your daily routine. In the evening, just give yourself one more minute and just repeat the steps above.

For now close this book and return tomorrow with just one more minute of yours from 24 hours ! and move on to the next chapter.

# 2. NEXT LEVEL

Hey! Feeling afresh? Ok I'll just have one minute of yours. Repeat the previous day workout just as same but try to increase the repetitions without disturbing any of your facial expressions.

Feeling pain? No problem, your body is adjusting to the pushups you are doing with the help of your wall. If the pain occurs in the evening, miss the evening workout. Keep this going on for 3-4 days and when you see the pain stops, it means your body has been accustomed to the pushups you do and is a clear indication from my side to move to the beginners level of the pushups all do in this world.

Every muscle in your body will now be forced to work and it's a great indication. Just ignore the pain and make sure you have to do lots and lots of gains.
Happy ! Not really? No problem dummy.

Have a glass of water in the morning and take out just one minute. Lay on the floor keeping your hands shoulder width apart and your body straight. Your legs should be as wide as your both the palms.

Now without disturbing your facial expression looking down to the ground make a move towards the ground only half way and do 3 times. Yeah ! I mean it 3 times.

The number of repetitions I am saying is so because it will not hurt you and side by side it help your muscles to adjust to your new hope to be daily routine. Now just move on with your daily chores and routine.

Come back tomorrow dummy. We will have some great time tomorrow

# 3 BEGINNER

Had a great sleep. No?. No one cares though. So, move into the same basic position of the pushup and do repetitions just increasing 1 repetition, means do it 4 times now. Over?

Come back again in the evening. Now do it 5 times. Not that tough? See now you can imagine the very first day you were not been able to give the time to pushups but now you are doing it 5 times(repetitions) and that too in only one minute. Probably in 30 seconds or less.

Just think you have to allot yourself a pretty damn 1minute. That's it. And I mean it after the completion of this book, you will be thanking yourself that you yourself was the only one criticizing yourself for not finding time. It is just simple as that you have to squeeze some time out.

Isn't that cool!. Sure it is. Now just increase your intake of pushups everyday just 1 more than the previous day. It is good if you want to do it in the evening otherwise if you still cannot find time it is still fine by me.

Ok lazy fella'. Keep it on for days. Just one minute to your life cycle of one day will just definitely give your body some tough time. Is that the case? Really? I don't think so.

Also day by day while moving your body down halfway, try to press it full just slightly above the ground. Try to do pushups as good they can be. It is not about the number of pushups but about how perfect you do each repetition

So just try not to overdo it.. If some pain is there, don't worry, body is accustoming.

Next chapter deals with why we do pushups?. What is the basic need to do? Why pushups are the basic form of exercise? The answer lies in the next chapter. Come again tomorrow to have some general knowledge about pushups.

Till then, have a good day !

# 4 WHY PUSHUPS?

So you must be following the regime and you must have think that why am I doing this stuff?

The answer lies here dummy. Pushups are just one of the most common and basic forms of exercises one could do in the given speculated time. Pushups are not only great for your chest but also it completely defines your abs, shoulder, triceps and torso.

And also one of the most important things, if you start early in your days, it could help you increase your height. I have that experience.

Pushups surely does add strength to your body. It shoots up your metabolism to a great extent. Also doing pushups one doesn't need excuses like there is no need of equipments and not time consuming. You can do pushups anywhere you like.

You just have to have a pair of hands!

There is a quote from New York Times which read "As a symbol of health and wellness, nothing surpasses the simple pushup. The pushup is the simple barometer of fitness. It tests the whole body engaging muscle groups to the arms, chest, abdomen, hips and legs. It requires the body to be taut like a plank with toes and palms on the floor.
The act of lifting and lowering one's entire weight is taxing even for the very fit."

# 5 VARIED FORMS(JUST FOR KNOWLEDGE)

**Knee push ups** – It will reduce your body weight to half. You can do the same exercise on your knees.
 Just keep your body straight, so please pay attention to correct body alignment as you perform your workout.

**Knuckle push ups** -These are not just for the hard-core push up folks. Some people experience wrist discomfort as they perform basic push ups, but by closing your hands and making a fist, your body weight ends up on your knuckles instead of your palms, thus avoiding the weight on your palms.
 **Note:** Please be sure to do this type of push up on a padded mat, plush carpet or even better a rolled up towel.

**Bench push ups** - You can also use a low bench or chair to support your arms while you perform either regular push ups or knee push ups. This type of push up allows you to really concentrate on the push up motion; all without the strain of the regular version.
 **Note:** Please be sure the bench or chair is stable and secure before you perform the push ups.

**Wall push ups(already explained)** - If all the above options are still too challenging, one final variation exists. The wall push up reduces the pressure on the arms, upper back and abs. The closer you stand to the wall, the easier they are to perform, but remember, it's still important to be aware of your body alignment as you perform the "wall" push up. As you gain strength and confidence, move your feet slightly further away from the wall to make the workout more challenging. Feel free to consider moving to the "bench" or "knee" style push ups once your initial strength has increased

# 6 INTERMEDIATE

Hi there ! Hope you are having a great time. It's pretty much shocking that you have gone this far in this book

So, I am hoping that you would be following the one minute schedule of pushups. I presume so. Now champ, we will head to some serious business about pushups.

Let's start now. Feeling afresh? No? never mind I'll still move on. Now since you have been doing pushups by increasing the repetitions, it would be tough for you me to increase the pushups intensity. You must be having some sort of elevated table in your house. Elevation should be about 3-6 inches. Not more than that. If not, then any type of elevation will do.

Just remember I am not forcing anyone. Now try to do pushups with the elevation starting with the maximum number and increasing the repetitions day by day. You can also balance yourself on a football and do pushups. It will work your abs too.

After 1 week of doing the monotonous routine of pushups on the elevation, now, move back to the basic pushup on the ground. Now just move your both the legs a bit closer than usual in the usual pushup position. Now go for the repetitions. Felt the pressure? Try to do the same number of pushups as before.

Try this position on elevation and master it!.

# 7 BETA VERSION

Hope you will be having some torrid time reading this book. Still I'll move on. Have some water and form the basic pushup on the ground. Now go for full depth touching the ground.
Now while touching the ground with your chest hold down for 3 seconds and then come up. Tough? Pretty much dummy.

Do this thing for around 1 week. After that do the reverse, that is hold yourself up for 3 seconds before going down. You can add variations to this like doing it both the ways, increasing the time hold.

Do this for some weeks. Now, you must be noticing some significant changes in your body. Ghosh! You have worked your at least every muscle. Sounds Good.

Now, since you are comfortable performing pushups just add some variations to them. Like, now close your both the legs while lying on the ground and do pushups, variations in the width of both the palms like lesser than the width of the shoulders or more than them.

You can try putting some weights on your back while performing pushups. Just remember do not over do the weights or you may hurt your back. Weights could be of any type from pillows to anything. Yeah I have tried everything.

One can also do pushups on an iron rod elevated above the ground and perform simple pushups doing variations whatever you want to.

Do the variations on the elevation, just combine every other thing that have been listed on one thing or the other. You can also work your triceps, by inching your palms closer to each other.

Or the next time you do pushups, just remember to shift your position of both the hands slightly towards backwards rather than normal position.

You can also put your one leg on top of the other in a criss-cross manner and do pushups, it works significantly. One position is that in which you while doing pushups put your one leg slightly wider than the other and consecutively on the other repetition put the other leg as same as the previous while putting back the first leg to its normal position.

Same thing you can do with your hands consecutively. In pushups you can add a dozens of other variations.

Just be more and more creative while performing pushups. No equipment is needed. Whatever comes to your mind try that and reveal to me also.

# 8 SOME MORE VARIATIONS

Start from the basic pushup position. Now while moving up, apply a sudden force such that your both the hands are in the air for a flash. These are known as extreme pushups. In this also you can manipulate as you want.

Lift one hand up while performing a basic pushup, such that a T shape is formed. Here also you can add weights to your hands. If one can do handstand, pushups can also be done on that.(only if you are a gymnast!).

Ever heard of the Hindu pushup originated from India. Yeah, it's one more sort of pushup where you have to form a inverted V shape of your body and then go down in the basic pushup position forming a U shape while coming up.

Put your both the legs against the wall and your both the hands touching the ground. Now perform the basic pushup, the Hindu pushup. Any variation will work.

One can also use on hand while doing pushups. Want to get tougher? Use your just 3 fingers(any of them) and perform the pushup adding varieties to it.

Assume a basic pushup position. Now while moving upwards stop in the middle and then go down. This will add to your bigger chests.

One can also do rotational pushups in which while performing the basic pushup while completed one rep move your hand upward while opening the face of your body sideways.
You can move your hand in the front, back or sideways. Just add variations.

On the leg variations, same thing to do as hands. Raise your leg simultaneously and consecutively upwards, sideways, broadening the width.

Just remember to slowly doing every variation while not hurting yourself.

# 9 YET MORE VARIATIONS

Form the basic pushup position. While going down, just reduce your speed and while coming up, be fast. You can do the vice versa.

Let's do the spider man pushup. In this you have to continue doing your pushups while simultaneously moving your one leg sideways just as the spider man crawls the wall.

Want some more variations? Reverse your hands and then perform pushups. You must have seen ROCKY starring Sylvester Stallone. In the ring he also does some variations with one hand pushups alternating between each repetition.

This is one kind of hell pushup. While moving up apply as mush force to perform a jackknife by touching you fingers to the toes in the mid air. Remember, you have to be extremely fit to do this.

Bruce Lee used to did two finger, single handed pushup. So, it is possible. Just keep on doing and doing and you will see the results all by yourself.

On a normal pushup position, while moving upwards, twist your mid torso sideways alternatively while moving your one leg at a time. It will help in maintaining your abs.

Put your both hands in the crossed motion slightly closer to each other. Now do basic pushups.

While stacking your both the legs against the wall apply every other variation you best described in this book and your innovations too. The resistance would be great for your upper strength. Try using a resistance band for performing the pushups if you have one, otherwise it is also fine.

Just add more and more variations whichever comes to your mind. Feel free to ask anything.

I think, in my first edition of pushups this is sufficient. While you master them, I'll be out soon with yet another form of exercise. I would love to hear from your side. Just mail me below at my mail id.

ashu3012199288@yahoo.com

# ABOUT THE AUTHOR

Currently I am a Software Developer. I have done my Bachelors in Technology from Electronics and Communication. I am a totally freak out guy about exercising. I will soon release my copies on other exercises. And yes, I have tried everything I have mentioned above. So, it's great to be a partner with you in performing those pushups. Hope to hear from you soon if you want to add some more things. Every reply would be appreciated.

www.ingramcontent.com/pod-product-compliance
Lightning Source LLC
Chambersburg PA
CBHW071351310526
45790CB00018B/1414